Reflexology

The Absolute Beginners Guide to Reflexology

by Linda Serpico

purposes solely, and is universal as so. The presentation of the information is without contract or any type of guarantee assurance.

The trademarks that are used are without any consent, and the publication of the trademark is without permission or backing by the trademark owner. All trademarks and brands within this book are for clarifying purposes only and are the owned by the owners themselves, not affiliated with this document.

Quick Note On Towdie Publishing

As a reward to you the reader we would like to let you know when other books like this are on FREE promotion. At Towdie, we work with writers around the world to consistently bring you high quality books in the fields of health, wellness and better living.

We also have an exciting series of books on spiritual and higher consciousness topics. When a new book is ready to publish we always give our loyal readers a chance to download the Kindle version for free. This is so that we can get your feedback on how to improve the book for future editions. This is why your Amazon review is very important to us.

If you would like to be part of our growing community of readers, please sign up to out mailing list and we will start sending you free books straight away.

Sign up here:
http://www.towdiebooks.com

Table of Content

Introduction

I want to thank you and congratulate you for downloading the book, *"Reflexology: The Absolute Beginners Guide to Reflexology"*.

This book contains proven steps and strategies on how to understand the basics of reflexology. This can serve as a guide for beginners in reflexology so they will know exactly what to do, what to prepare and where to begin.

This book contains a step-by-step guide on how beginners can easily perform three of the most popular types of reflexology – the foot, hand and face reflexology. This also has many tips and contains the right techniques to use for each type.

Thanks again for buying this book, I hope you enjoy it!

Chapter 1 - The Basics about Reflexology

Do you believe that the body has the ability to heal itself? This is among its many wonders that many people tend to ignore, especially these days when there seems to be a medicine or facility that can cure almost all kinds of health problems. There are times when it is better to prove this claim. You can allow time to heal your wounds naturally or learn how to facilitate an alternative kind of medicine, such as reflexology.

Reflexology, aside from being one form of alternative medicine, is known as a natural healing art. It follows the idea that the body has reflexes in the hand and feet that match every part of your body. You will need to find these reflexes, stimulate and apply pressure to promote the function and get rid of any aches that each of your body part is suffering from.

If you will only take time to observe, your feet and hands are actually more sensitive than how you perceive them to be. These body parts can detect movement, weight alignment, stretch and pressure.

How Reflexology Works

This kind of alternative medicine is best administered by a practitioner who has undergone training about the pressure points in the body. You can also do this on your own, with the help of certain tools designed to help you easily locate these pressure points. You will then need to learn how to use your thumbs and hands to stimulate these points and address the body parts that correspond to these.

What it is not?

While reflexology is widely used around the world to complement other treatment methods for different health problems, it is never intended to cure or diagnose any disorder. It is commonly done as a preventive measure, especially in health conditions that include anxiety, diabetes, kidney failure, PMS, asthma and migraine.

This method of alternative medicine now receives increased attention from various countries around the world. In Denmark, some studies proved that the application of reflexology resulted in fewer sick leaves and absences from employees. The country employs reflexologists in their companies and municipalities since the beginning of the 90s. It has increased the level of productivity of employees that equates to economic savings for employers.

Understanding the Reflexology Points and Areas

There are points and areas that are situated in the hands, feet and face that correspond to different body organs and parts. This is the first thing that you have to learn in the practice – to locate where these points and areas are and what body part do they correspond. Even the professionals have used maps of reflex points that are now available in different forms and are made from various materials.

While some practitioners explain the minor reflex points differently, most of them agree when it comes to the major reflex points in the body. When you go to a professional, you will be asked what is bothering you so that he can locate the points that correspond to your concern. He will work on your whole body before focusing on your problem areas.

If you are in a hurry, but in obvious distress, you will likely be given a relaxation session. In this case, the reflexologist will work on your ears until your nerves have calmed down. The core of the practice is to release the stress or congestion in your nervous system and attain the right energy balance.

Reflexology versus Other Forms of Therapies

Reflexology is often compared and related to two other forms of alternative medicine - acupuncture and acupressure. All these therapies work by stimulating the essential points in the body to release the needed energy and try to alleviate whatever the patient is suffering from. There may be certain similarities, but some of the pressure points that are utilized in acupuncture and acupressure do not coincide with the reflex points that comprise the reflexology map.

In acupressure, a practitioner traces more than 800 reflex points that run throughout the body and are situated along the meridians. The latter is described as the thin and long energy lines that run across the whole body.

Reflexology is also often confused with another form of alternative treatment, which is massage. Both methods utilize touch, but in different approaches. Massage relaxes the muscles by doing certain techniques, such as kneading, stroke, tapping and friction.
Reflexology does not involve the techniques that are employed in a massage. It instead utilizes what is known as micro-movements. Instead of big and forceful movements like in a massage, a practitioner will walk and hook the reflex points using the thumb or finger until your body responds to the motion. If a massage therapist works from the outer part of your body to address what's bothering you from the inside, the opposite is applied by a reflexologist.

The latter stimulates the nervous system by working from the points that are found inside your body to affect and work on its outer areas. You will remain fully clothed during a reflexology session, which is not always true with massage because the therapist has to use oils or ointments to work on the outer areas of your body.

A Brief Look on Its History

Its origin is really hard to track because reflexology has been practiced since the ancient times. It is believed that it was passed through generations via an oral tradition. There were traces in history where pictographs used to practice this method can be proven. For example, there were imprints of feet that were found in an Egyptian tomb of Ankhamor in 2330 BC.

A book that was considered a classic in China, entitled the Yellow Emperor's Classic of Internal Medicine, has a chapter dedicated to the points that are found on the feet and how these points affect the whole body. The book was written in 1,000 BC.

In the US, William H. Fitzgerald, MD is often referred to as the father of this kind of alternative medicine. It was due to the book that he released in 1917 about the 10 vertical zones that run throughout the body. It also tackled how one can locate an injury and relieve its pain by applying pressure to the right points and areas.

Many doctors and practitioners continue to study and work with this method through time. For one, Dr. Shelby Riley expanded the studies conducted by Dr. Fitzgerald. Dr. Riley was able to come up with the detailed map of the reflex points in the hands and feet.
Dr. Riley worked closely with a physiotherapist, Eunice Ingham, who continued with the research and found out

that the most responsive and sensitive to the pressure points are the feet. Ingham created the foot maps that are still utilized up until now. She also designed a reflexology chart that remains useful and popular to date. This chart was refined by Ingham's nephew, Dwight Byers, who works at the International Reflexology Institute.

The map of the reflex points in the ear was recorded by Dr. Paul Nogier in 1957. The map has since undergone expansion and improvement, and is now being utilized by many practitioners and enthusiasts.

Chapter 2 - Therapeutic Effects of Reflexology

How does reflexology affect the body? How do you benefit from the process of stimulating your reflex areas?

1. Neurophysiological benefits

The nervous system benefits the most from the pressure that is applied to the feet and hands as you undergo the therapeutic touch of reflexology. There are studies that are being conducted to prove the relationship between the nervous system and the endocrine and immune system.

For now, the obvious effects of reflexology that fall under this category include the normalization of heart rate, and feeling more relaxed and happy. This also boosts your energy levels and causes you to have quality sleep. This makes you feel good about yourself in general. It can also improve your digestion and respiration, and reduce the levels of your stress and anxiety.

2. Improved vascular and lymphatic circulation

There was a research in Japan that was done in the 90s, which proved that this kind of alternative medicine can boost the blood circulation in the legs. This is especially helpful to patients who are immobile or have difficulty walking or moving around. A therapeutic foot massage has the ability to lower both the systolic and diastolic blood pressure. This can also help in lowering a patient's pulse rate.

3. Touch

Touch is an effective therapy to people of all ages, from babies to the elderlies. It is believed that a simple touch can heal. This is evident with the different massage techniques done to soothe and calm newborns and babies. There are also lots of nursing homes that make touch therapy a part of how the staff and nurses take care of their patients.

Have you ever experienced feeling so low and sad, but a simple touch on the hand or a hug from a loved one, eases your sadness away? Touch can heal. It gives you the feeling that someone cares. It goes through a person's core. It conveys a lot of emotions, such as warmth, love, trust and respect.

4. Balances your energy

The pressure applied to the different points of your body helps in making you experience the optimum state of homeostasis. The massage unblocks the pathways and balances the energy in your whole system.

5. Makes you experience ultimate relaxation

The pressure applied to the reflex points in your body relaxes the organs that correspond to these points. The feeling of relaxation comes from the smoother blood and energy flow in your system. Your nerves also calm down and in the end, heal your being.

6. Healing effects

Reflexology has other positive effects that many people have already benefited from. This helps in relieving migraines and headaches. It eases away your body pains and reduces inflammation. This also reduces the symptoms of PMT and kidney problems. It aids in lowering your blood sugar levels and helps in improving your overall digestive health. This also reduces the restlessness that a person who has dementia often experiences. This is also good for the thyroid and gall bladder.

Chapter 3 - Important Pointers and Techniques

It is easy to learn reflexology. It will help a lot to print a reflexology chart that you can use as a guide as you follow the techniques that beginners like you can easily perform. The next chapters will teach you about the basics on how to perform reflexology on the foot, face and hand. Before you learn about the specifics, here are some important things that you ought to know about this kind of alternative medicine.

1. It is not recommended to perform the massage to people who have been bedridden for more than 24 hours. If they have only recuperated from certain illnesses, their pain tolerance is still low. If they will ask you to go on with the massage, be extra gentle. Frequently pause and ask if they don't get hurt by the pressure that you are using.

2. An ideal session lasts for more than 30 minutes, depending on the age and body built of the patient. If you are attending to an ill patient, an elderly or someone who is still young, it is not recommended to go beyond 30 minutes.

3. It is best to do the whole body massage instead of focusing on specific pressure points, depending on the health problems of the patient. Perform the whole treatment and spend more time in applying pressure to where the pressure points of the patient's health concerns are situated.

4. When learning how to perform reflexology, it is recommended to begin with the foot. You will

likely find more written studies and researches about this type of reflexology, since this is widely done in many countries across the globe.
When you have already perfected the techniques, you can easily perform reflexology on other parts of the body.

5. It is not ideal to use massage oils and creams in performing reflexology. These materials may help in relaxing and calming the nerves of the patient, but these can make it harder for you to exert pressure on your touch. The skin will be slippery. If you want to use these, it is best to apply the oils and creams at the end of the session. Allow the smell and the effects of these products to linger on the patient to help him further relax after the massage.
Instead of oils and creams, you can use a talcum or baby powder when you are performing the massage. The powder will absorb the oils from the patient's body, which will help you easily apply the needed pressure. Simply sprinkle the powder to the patient's feet and hands before you begin with the process. You can also choose a powder with a nice scent that can make your patient relax throughout the massage.

6. If the patient is diabetic, ask him to check his blood sugar before you begin and when you are done with the session. A person may experience a severe rise or drop of his blood sugar levels when undergoing this kind of alternative medicine.

7. You have to learn the right techniques that you should use in applying pressure on different body parts. For example, the best technique that can effectively work on the surface of the feet is thumb walking. You can use a circular motion of the index

finger in massaging the hands to make the pressure firmer and deeper.

8. Both the person who is administering reflexology and the receiver must be comfortable during the whole session.. You can let your patient sit or lie, depending on his preference. If you are doing the massage, do it in angles that you are most comfortable with. It will reflect on your touch if you feel uneasy or awkward. In performing the techniques, it is best not to bend over and never put pressure on your knees.

9. People react differently when undergoing a reflexology session. Some simply enjoy the process and try to relax while others may fall asleep. There are also patients who show physical responses during or after the massage. These responses include burping, coughing, spasms and farting. Some also experience tiredness and lack of energy after the have undergone their first session. You can minimize such reactions by reminding the patient to drink lots of water before and after the session. You must also keep a bottle of water handy during the massage and tell your patient to drink whenever he wants to.

Chapter 4 - Foot Reflexology

The first thing that you have to learn in administering foot reflexology is the thumb walking technique. You can do this for a long period without causing strain to your hand. The concept is easy. You will let your thumb walk forward by bending and unbending the finger.

The first thing that you need to accomplish is to practice your thumbs. Look at the upper part of your two thumbs by placing the two next to each other and examining them closely. Roll the top parts of your thumbs until the nails are almost touching. The part where the two thumbs almost touch will be used in the massage.

Use a pen in practicing the technique. Hold it with your hand. Use the thumb of your other hand and touch the pen with the part that was described above. Bend the thumb, allow it to straighten and repeat the process. As you do this, make sure that the pen does not move and your thumb stays in contact with it. This is where the pressure will come from.

You will exert pressure whenever the thumb is straightened and let the finger move forward as it bends. Start slow. As you get the hang of it, you can do the technique at a faster rate. You can also practice this at similar surfaces, such as on tables and chairs. This technique gives a thorough treatment to the entire feet.

Start with the Foot Reflexology

Always begin the session on the right foot. Print out a diagram of foot reflexology to make it easier for you to locate the pressure points in the feet. Here are the steps to get this done.

1. Relax the foot by massaging it all over in a slow manner. Move from the toes to the heel. Do this for 30 seconds or until you feel that the muscles start to relax and loosen up.

   Cup the spine area of the foot with the palm of your one hand and hold the bottom with the thumb of your other hand. Perform a gentle twist by slowly wringing your hands away from one another. Do this for 30 seconds.

2. Start with the thumb walking action in the spine of the foot. Work from the heel to toes, then down from the toes back to the heel. Do the action from the left to the right direction of the spine until you have covered the entire foot.

3. Hold the big toe and gently rotate it. Do this action to the rest of the toes until you are done with the smallest one. As you rotate, try to stretch the base joint that holds the toe to the foot. This motion works on the bones in your head. This is believed to be effective in relieving headaches.

4. Find the meridian points on the toes, which are situated at the end of the toes, except for the middle finger. You will then apply pressure on the meridian point of each toe by making a circular movement. Move the toe clockwise for 10 seconds and counter-clockwise for another 10 seconds. Start with the big toe and work until you are finished with the smallest.

5. Begin the thumb-walk exercise on the toes. Move upwards, from the base to the tip, following a straight line. Do this action until you are done with all sides of all toes. The pressure has to be solid, yet gentle.

Take note that there are certain people whose toes are quite sensitive. You must first experiment with the pressure and ask them their preference. Never lose the firmness in the pressure. It will tickle your patient if you will just gently apply pressure.

6. Perform the massage on the ball of the foot, which is referred to as the chest region. Do this in a gentle upward motion, downwards and in an angular motion until the entire region is covered.

7. Work on the top and back of the foot. Begin from the toes to the ankle then from the right to the left side of the foot.

8. Look at your printed diagram and look where the waistline is located. This is the thinnest part at the bottom part of the foot and the location may differ from person to person. Thumb walk on the entire area, which corresponds to the liver and stomach.

9. You will now perform the thumb walk in the area that is situated in between the pelvic region and the waistline.

10. Perform the massage on the pelvic area, which corresponds to the sciatic nerve. Do the action from the left side going to the right then all the way up and at the back of the heel.

11. When you are done, massage the entire foot in a relaxing and gentle manner for a minute.

You are now done with the right foot. Repeat the steps, but this time, work on the left foot of your patient.

Make sure that you have drinking water on hand during

the session. Make the patient drink a glass of water before you begin. This will help the blood to get rid of the toxins from the body. Advise your patient to continue drinking water for the whole day after the session.

Chapter 5 - Face Reflexology

Face reflexology can be self-administered, but you can also perform this to other people. Before you begin, make sure that you have printed out a face reflexology chart to make it easier for you to locate which areas to work on.

Familiarize yourself with the 15 points in the face. Applying pressure to these points will boost a person's blood circulation and this is a great way to relax. This is typically given to those who want to take a breather and recharge from all the stresses that they are constantly facing.

You can use your index finger or thumb to apply pressure on the reflex points on the face. Gently push the finger on the pressure point and rotate it without lifting the finger. Do the action on the same spot, 30 seconds in a clockwise motion and another 30 seconds in the opposite direction.

In performing this kind of reflexology, it is best that the person who is undergoing the treatment is seated. The shoulders and head must be fully supported. Perform the action behind your patient to make it more comfortable for you to move.

Here are the steps on how to get this done:

1. Stimulate the reflex points in the face one at a time. Follow a diagram and work on the points in sequential order. Work on the whole face first before you focus and repeat applying pressure to any specific points.

2. Tap the part under the eyes using the tip of the

fingers of your two hands. The tapping has to be gentle. Tap from the nose to the ears. Rub the jaw line, still using two hands, from the top part of the ears, all the way to the chin. Put your index fingers on the chin and begin rubbing this part for about 15 seconds. Now move the fingers from the chin to the edges of the mouth, until you reach the cheeks. Rub the cheeks in a circular manner for 30 seconds.

Move your fingers to the nose, forehead then work on the two eyebrows by rubbing your fingers in an outward motion. Pull the fingers upwards until you have reached the hairline. Rub this part then work on the scalp. You can spend as much time as you want in this area because this is extremely relaxing.

3. To maximize the benefits of this form of reflexology, remind your patient about the importance of water. You have to let your patient drink water before the session and the succeeding hours after that. The patient has to take a break and rest after the session is over.

Chapter 6 - Hand Reflexology

The techniques that are employed in hand reflexology are different from the methods used in giving foot reflexology. The hands are flexible and the pressure points are found deep under the skin. This means that you have to exert more effort in pressing and holding the pressure to stimulate the points.

Sit across a table from the person who will receive the treatment. Give your patient a towel that he can place under his hands to offer support and comfort. Begin the session with a relaxation exercise. Bear in mind that the hand reflexes are deeper than any of the pressure points in the body. Push the spot using your thumb. Apply a solid, but firm pressure. Rotate your thumb in a circular manner for five seconds. Move the thumb to your next target spot and repeat the same steps for another five seconds.

Now that you have relaxed the muscles and nerves in the hands, you can begin with the hand reflexology by following these steps:

Make sure that you first work on the right hand, finish the entire hand before you move to the left one.

1. Apply a little amount of baby oil around the wrist of the right hand. Massage this area using a big outward motion using your thumbs. Work your thumbs until you reach the palm of the patient. Massage the inside part of the palm and slowly, move towards the edges. Repeat the process in a slow manner for 30 seconds. Turn the hand over. Using your thumb, begin pushing each knuckle

from the bottom, to the wrist.

Make sure that you remain gentle because the action can be painful when you apply too much pressure. Hold a finger at a time. Give each finger a gentle twist from side to side. Gently squeeze the hand to end the relaxation exercise. You can remove the oil by tapping it with a tissue or towel. Perform the same actions on the other hand.

2. Find the meridians that are located in the hands. Work on each meridian in a circular manner, spending five seconds in a clockwise motion and five seconds in a counter clockwise direction. This is how you will stimulate the meridians including the lung, heart constrictor, colon, heart, small intestine and the triple burner.
   The triple burner meridian does not correspond to any body organ. This pertains to the three major cavities that contain the body organs within. When you stimulate this meridian, you can boost the balance all throughout your patient's system.

3. Work on the fingers that correspond to the organs and senses from the neck up. Work from the top part of the thumb of the right hand. Gently, move in the direction of the base of the thumb. Cover all areas of the thumb using the same movement from the top to the base. Work slowly until you have stimulated the whole thumb.

   Repeat the process for each of the fingers on the hand that you are working on. Work on the part under the little finger. This is beneficial in relieving minor shoulder pains. Pay attention and cover all the skin from the core to the outside areas.

4. Work on the palm that corresponds to the body's

torso. Lay the hand of the patient on the table with the palm facing upwards. Apply pressure on the soft skin under the fingers, moving downwards then up and sideways. Do the same procedure to the center of the palm. Spend more time working on the base of the thumb and the outer areas of the hand, making sure that you don't forget any soft padding situated between the wrist and the palm. This part corresponds to the digestive area and the spine. Rub the wrist from left to right and repeat, but this time, move in the opposite direction.

5. Turn the hand until the palm is faced down so that you can work on the back of the hand. This part is extra sensitive, so be gentle in applying pressure. Begin working on the knuckles to the wrist until you are done with all areas. You can then work on the wrist and the wrist bone.

6. Do all the above mentioned steps on the left hand.

You can end the process by doing a round of relaxation exercises for each hand. You can apply a cream or oil for this purpose. Work on the knuckles to the wrist of each hand for 30 seconds. Perform a rubbing motion around the wrist for 15 seconds. Make sure to cover all areas of the hand. You can add more oil or cream if you think that it is necessary. Wring out each finger before you end the exercise for each hand. All your movements need to be slow and gentle. Repeat the process with the other hand.

Hand reflexology is specifically helpful in getting rid of headaches. Similar to the other forms of reflexology, water is an important element to make the process effective. Make the patient drink water before the session. Advise him to drink water during the session whenever he feels like it. It is also important that your patient continues to drink more water for the next 24 hours and get sufficient rest.

Final Notes about Reflexology

You can take advantage of training programs to give you a full coverage on what you need to know about this kind of alternative medicine. You can take this action if you want to get proper certification so you can do this professionally. If you only want to learn the proper techniques that you can perform to yourself and to your loved ones, it is enough to follow the guides given in this book and learn how to read reflexology charts that you can download online.

Reflexology is a tool that encourages the body to heal on its own. The process is not intended to heal. Instead, it stimulates the different areas and pivotal points in your body to start working and meet their potential to heal. The good thing about the process is that it is safe. It is also quite relaxing and enjoyable.

You can give a session or two to your loved one as a gift. You can also pamper yourself by spending some time working on your own pressure points. Keep doing the techniques and read more about the process after you have perfected what you have learned. This is the only way for you to get better at performing this to other people and administering it to yourself.

There are a few cautions that you have to bear in mind to ensure that the process is safe and comfortable for both you and your patient.

- Give sufficient water to your patient before, during and after the session.
- If you are using scented candles to set the room's

ambience, remember that scented candles can produce too much scent and heat. Use the type with a mild scent and make sure that the room has proper air ventilation.

- It is best to do the massage in a dimly-lit room. It helps in relaxing your patient. If you can't find this kind of space, you can put an eye mask to your patient to achieve the same effect.

Conclusion

Thank you again for nuying this book!

I hope this book was able to help you to understand the basics about reflexology and how to get started with it.

The next step is to follow the guides and start practicing. In time, you will get better with it and you may find yourself looking for more advanced lessons about reflexology.

Finally, if you enjoyed this book, then I'd like to ask you for a favour, would you be kind enough to leave a review for this book on Amazon? It'd be greatly appreciated!

Please leave a review for this book on Amazon!

Thank you and good luck!

If you enjoyed this book you may wish to check out this book also by the author:

"PALMISTRY: How To Read Palms For Beginners"

by Linda Serpico

We hold secrets to our life in the palm of our hand. This may sound too good to be true.Read further into this subject in this captivating and thorough book and perhaps you will change your mind. You will start to understand the world of Palmistry and why many people from cultures around the world all through out time have looked to the palm for the secrets to life.

Find out more about this book here:
http://www.amazon.com/PALMISTRY-Beginners-Palmistry-chiromancy-divination-ebook/dp/B0180TX3KG

Learn More About The Towdie Publishing Catalogue

Towdie Publishing is a small independent publisher focused on bringing together the best information on spiritual and higher consciousness subjects and also on alternative and vibrant health and wellness.

We are constantly working with writers around the world to bring to you the leading edge of information in each field. We have a mission to help heal the world and bring it back into harmony through providing people with the knowledge and education they need to transform their lives for the better.

We want to thank you for supporting our mission by buying this book. We value your time and attention and hope that this book has brought to you information that will bring positive transformation in your life.

If you have enjoyed this book you may also wish to look to some of the other best selling books in our catalogue. Please check out some of our other books below:

Spiritual And Higher Consciousness Catalogue

"KUNDALINI: The Secret To Unlocking Your Inner Spiritual Power"

by Roderick Towdie

You're about to discover how to safely start working towards a permanent awakening of Kundalini. The awakening of this mystical energy, spoken of in secret for thousands of years, is the goal of meditation traditions around the world. This book will take you on an exciting introductory journey to unlocking your secret spiritual power.

Find out more here:
http://www.amazon.com/gp/product/B017O3U9TM

"CHAKRAS: How To Feel , Grow And Balance Your Chakras"

by Dan Godchild

You're about to discover how to safely start working on your Chakras, developing them and opening them. Why would you want to walk this path? Working with your Chakras is the key to opening yourself to a new life. Grow a new sense of strength and balance in the world and release negative emotions that stand in your way to peace and enlightenment in this life. This book can give you the key to beginning your journey to working with your Chakras.

Find out more here:
http://www.amazon.com/CHAKRAS-beginners-balancing-meditation-explained-ebook/dp/B0181FBN1K

"VISION BOARD: Create The Life You Want Using A Vision Board"

by Devan Skywisdom

Master manifestor Devan Skywisdom was recently commissioned with the challenge of succeeding where other writers have, so far, failed. You see, there is simply no book out there that brings together the subject of Vision Boards so clearly, so powerfully and in such an easy and entertaining manner. This guide is designed in mind for the earnest seeker looking for perhaps the first time into the mysterious world of Vision Board creation.

Find out more about this book here:
http://www.amazon.com/VISION-BOARD-Create-attraction-affirmations-ebook/dp/B01833W95O

"FASTING: The Truth About The Most Powerful And Ancient Healing Method Of All"

Linda Serpico

by James Horran

Few people realise the powerful healing potential that lies dormant within their body. Our modern lives filled with stress and drama and accompanied by a modern diet filled with processed and hard to digest food leaves the body with little time and energy to do the healing it requires for total wellness. Fasting in a controlled environment can bring incredible benefits to a persons life. Not only can illnesses and and aches and pains that have plagued people for years completely dissappear but a new sense of purpose and clarity can dawn on a person.

Find out more in this book: http://www.amazon.com/FASTING-Powerful-Ancient-intermittent-fastting-ebook/dp/B017P7Z69A

"HYPNOSIS: Instant Hypnosis Secrets You Need To Know"

by Dane Xander

This book will show you how it is possible for anyone to use hypnotic techniques to change their own behavior and influence how other people acts. At the same time, you would also learn how to protect yourself from hypnosis.

Find out more about this book here: http://www.amazon.com/HYPNOSIS-Hypnosis-hypnosis-hypnotize-hypnotism-ebook/dp/B019TKWS4C

"MENTALISM: The Absolute Beginners Guide To Mentalism"

by Dane Xander

You Can Develop The Ability To Blow Peoples Minds With Mentalism! This book contains proven steps and strategies on how to understand the secrets that professional mentalists use. This book will also show you how you can perform mentalism tricks, expand your perception skills and be able to make use of basic mind manipulation strategies.

Find out more about this book here: http://www.amazon.com/MENTALISM-Beginners-Mentalism-mentalism-hypnotism-ebook/dp/B019D7KQXG

"LAW OF ATTRACTION: How To Attract Your Soulmate Using The Law Of Attraction"

by Linda Jameson

The Law of Attraction is not an entirely new concept. Ancient societies have been following its ideas and practices. It has only gained renewed attention because more and more people are discovering that the Law of Attraction works and that it can help in various aspects of life, even in the quest for a soulmate.

Find out more about this book here: http://www.amazon.com/LAW-ATTRACTION-Soulmate-Attraction-attraction-ebook/dp/B019IYQJCG

Health and Wellness Catalogue

"METABOLISM: How To Eat To Optimise Your Metabolism, Lose Weight And Get In The Best Shape Of Your Life"

by Ronald Towdie

This book hopes to debunk some of the myths about our metabolism and teach you the secrets to eat well to boost your metabolism and improve your health. You will also understand how to incorporate more raw food in your life to supercharge your metabolism. It also includes some helpful tips that can enable you to improve your metabolism and a lot more.

Find out more about this book here: http://www.amazon.com/METABOLISM-Optimize-Metabolism-metabolic-metabolism-ebook/dp/B016E98PVG

"PALEO DIET: 17 Reasons To Avoid The Paleo Diet"

by Ronald Towdie

In recent years the Paleo Diet has became a craze that has swept the nation. But does this diet really have the health benefits that it claims to have? Before you try this diet you should read this important book to help you consider whether this is the best choice for you and your family.

Find out more here: http://www.amazon.com/PALEO-DIET-Reasons-beginners-cookbook-ebook/dp/B019TLIWXM

"CALISTHENICS: Simple Bodyweight Exercises To Build Strength, Size And Balance Without Going To The Gym"

by Towdie Jones

Discover the Calisthenics book that gives you two detailed and complete 28 day routines to lead you to strength, flexibility and total wellness! You're about to discover how to immediately start incorporating Calisthenics training into your life. Benefit from this books detailed description of all of the classic Calisthenics exercises and the two complete 28 day routines that you can start working on.

Find out more about this book here:
http://www.amazon.com/CALISTHENICS-Bodyweight-Exercises-calisthenics-bodyweight-ebook/dp/B0180TJN3W

"RAW FOOD: Lazy Man's Guide To Raw Food Success"

by Ronnie Smith

Is there an easy way to success with a raw food diet? Find out more in this clear and simple book. If you are looking for clear, simple and no nonsense advice on thriving on a raw food lifestyle this is the book to get!

Find out more here: http://www.amazon.com/Raw-Food-Guide-Success-801010-ebook/dp/B0173S5MLI

"RAW VEGAN: How To Be A Raw Vegan Smart Ass"

by Ronnie Smith

Are you a raw vegan that hates getting all the same questions over and over again? If you would like some great one liners, smart ass answers and awesome replies to the most common questions asked of people eating a raw vegan diet then check out this book.

Find out more about this book here: http://www.amazon.com/Raw-Vegan-Compilation-Funniest-Questions-ebook/dp/B015ASXJ68

To sign up to our list and be notified when our upcoming books are on FREE promotion, please join us at our website here:

http://www.towdiebooks.com

Thank you!

Made in the USA
Lexington, KY
06 May 2016